Juicing For Diabetes

"A Step-by-Step Guide to Lowering Your Blood Sugar and Boosting Your Health"

PETER MILLER

Introduction

Chapter 1

Understanding Diabetes and Juicing

Chapter 2

Getting Started with Juicing for Diabetes

Choosing the Right Juicer

Selecting the Best Fruits and Vegetables for Juicing

Preparing Fruits and Vegetables for Juicing

Chapter 3

Essential Nutrients for Diabetes Management

Chapter 4

Juicing Recipes for Diabetes Management

Chapter 5

Creating a Juicing Routine for Diabetes Management

Incorporating Juicing into Your Daily Routine

When to Juice and How Often

Tracking the Effects of Juicing on Blood Sugar Levels

Chapter 6

Juicing for Weight Loss and Diabetes Management

The Link Between Weight Loss and Diabetes Management

Using Juicing as Part of a Healthy Weight Loss Program

Tips and Tricks for Creating Low-Calorie, High-Nutrient Juices

Chapter 7

Overcoming Common Juicing Challenges

Time Constraints

Budget Concerns

Juicer Malfunctions

Unappetizing Juices

Chapter 8

Integrating Juicing into a Comprehensive Diabetes Management Plan

Integrating Juicing into a Comprehensive Diabetes Management Plan

Creating a Sustainable and Effective Diabetes Management Plan

Chapter 9

Juicing Beyond Diabetes Management

Benefits of Juicing for Overall Health

Recipes for Juices that Promote Overall Health and Wellness

Tips for Using Juicing as Part of a Broader Health and Wellness Routine

Chapter 10

The Power of Juicing for Diabetes Management

Introduction

Diabetes is a chronic condition that affects millions of people worldwide, and managing blood sugar levels can be a daily struggle for those who suffer from it. Although there are medications available to help control diabetes, lifestyle changes such as diet and exercise can also play a critical role in managing the disease.

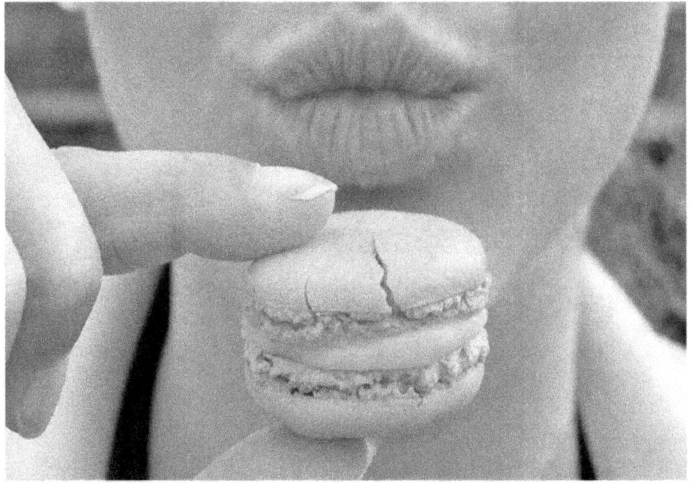

One of the most effective and natural ways to manage diabetes is through juicing. Juicing offers a convenient and delicious way to consume a variety of fruits and vegetables that are packed with essential vitamins, minerals, and antioxidants that can help lower blood sugar levels and boost overall health.

This book, "Juicing for Diabetes: A Step-by-Step Guide to Lowering Your Blood Sugar and Boosting Your Health," is designed to provide readers with a comprehensive guide to juicing for diabetes management. The book offers step-by-step instructions on how to create delicious and nutritious juices that are specifically tailored to help manage diabetes.

In addition to providing a range of delicious juicing recipes, the book also provides important information on the nutritional benefits of different fruits and vegetables, as well as tips and tricks for getting the most out of your juicing routine.

Whether you're newly diagnosed with diabetes or have been managing the disease for years, this book is an essential resource for anyone looking to take control of their health and lower their blood sugar levels through the power of juicing. With "Juicing for Diabetes," you'll discover a whole new world of delicious and healthy juices that can help you manage your diabetes and improve your overall health and wellbeing.

Chapter 1

Understanding Diabetes and Juicing

Diabetes is a chronic condition that affects the way your body processes blood sugar (glucose), which is the primary source of energy for your cells. There are two main types of diabetes: type 1 and type 2. Type 1 diabetes is an autoimmune disorder in which the body's immune system attacks and destroys the cells in the pancreas that produce insulin, a hormone that regulates blood sugar levels. Type 2 diabetes is a condition in which the body becomes resistant to insulin or doesn't produce enough of it.

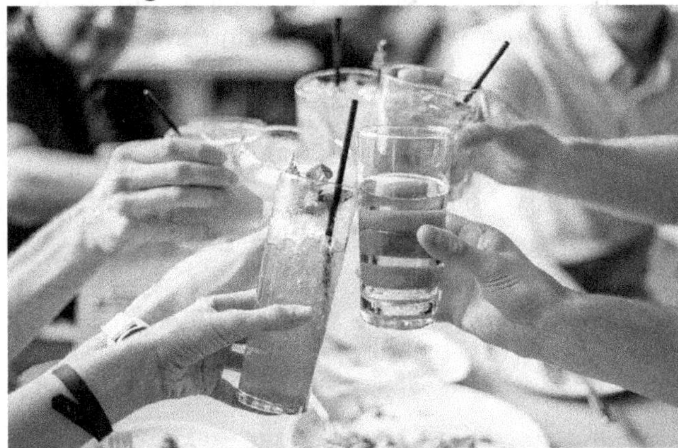

Both types of diabetes can lead to high blood sugar levels, which can cause a range of health complications over time, including nerve damage, kidney damage, and cardiovascular disease. Managing diabetes is essential for preventing these complications, and lifestyle changes such as diet and exercise can play a critical role in diabetes management.

One effective and natural way to manage diabetes is through juicing. Juicing involves extracting the juice from fruits and vegetables, leaving behind the pulp and fiber. This allows you to consume a concentrated source of nutrients and antioxidants that can help lower blood sugar levels and improve overall health.

The benefits of juicing for diabetes are numerous. First and foremost, juicing allows you to consume a variety of fruits and vegetables that are packed with essential vitamins and minerals, as well as antioxidants that can help lower inflammation and improve insulin sensitivity. Juicing also allows you to consume a larger quantity of fruits and vegetables than you might otherwise be able to eat in a single sitting, making it a convenient way to get the nutrients you need to manage diabetes.

Juicing can also help regulate blood sugar levels by providing a source of carbohydrates that are absorbed more slowly than those found in processed foods and sugary drinks. This can help prevent spikes in blood sugar levels and provide sustained energy throughout the day.

In addition to the nutritional benefits of juicing, it can also be a tasty and enjoyable way to manage diabetes. Juices can be customized to suit your tastes and preferences, and there are endless combinations of fruits and vegetables that can be used to create delicious and nutritious juices.

However, it's important to note that not all juices are created equal when it comes to managing diabetes. Some juices, particularly those that are high in sugar, can actually cause blood sugar levels to spike. It's essential to choose the right fruits and vegetables for juicing and to pay attention to the sugar content of the juices you consume.

In summary, juicing can be a powerful tool for managing diabetes. By providing a concentrated source of essential nutrients and antioxidants, juicing can help lower blood sugar levels and improve overall health. However, it's important to choose the right fruits and vegetables for juicing and to pay attention to the sugar content of the juices you consume. In the following chapters, we'll explore how to get started with juicing, the essential nutrients for diabetes management, and a range of delicious and nutritious juicing recipes tailored specifically for diabetes management.

Chapter 2

Getting Started with Juicing for Diabetes

Juicing is a simple and effective way to consume a variety of fruits and vegetables that can help manage diabetes. However, getting started with juicing can be intimidating, especially if you've never juiced before. In this chapter, we'll provide a comprehensive guide to getting started with juicing for diabetes, including choosing the right juicer, selecting the best fruits and vegetables for juicing, and preparing them for juicing.

Choosing the Right Juicer

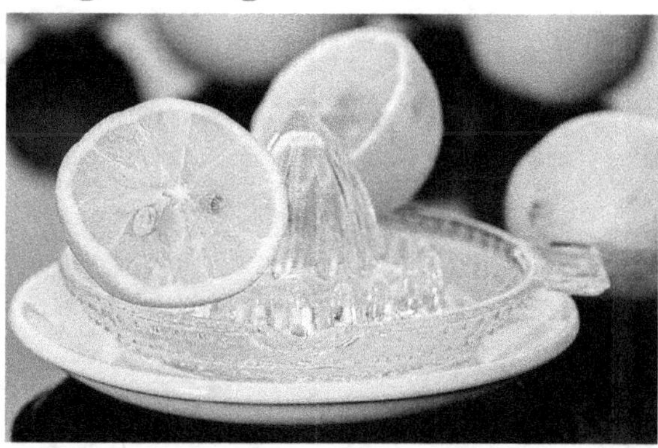

The first step in getting started with juicing is choosing the right juicer for your needs. There are two main types of juicers: centrifugal juicers and masticating juicers.

Centrifugal juicers work by spinning fruits and vegetables at high speeds to extract the juice. These juicers are typically more affordable and easier to use than masticating juicers, but they also tend to produce juice with less pulp and fiber, which can be important for diabetes management.

Masticating juicers, on the other hand, work by slowly crushing and grinding fruits and vegetables to extract the juice. These juicers are generally more expensive than centrifugal juicers but produce juice that is higher in fiber and nutrients.

When choosing a juicer for diabetes management, it's important to consider the quality of the juice as well as the cost and ease of use. A masticating juicer may be the better choice for those who prioritize nutrition and fiber, while a centrifugal juicer may be a better choice for those on a budget or who want a more convenient juicing experience.

Selecting the Best Fruits and Vegetables for Juicing

Once you've chosen a juicer, the next step is selecting the best fruits and vegetables for juicing. When it comes to managing diabetes, it's important to choose fruits and vegetables that are low in sugar and high in fiber and nutrients.

Leafy greens such as spinach, kale, and collard greens are excellent choices for juicing, as they are low in sugar and high in fiber and nutrients. Other good options include broccoli, celery, cucumber, carrots, and beets.

When selecting fruits for juicing, it's important to choose those that are low in sugar and high in fiber. Some good options include berries, apples, pears, and citrus fruits such as lemons and limes.

It's also important to consider the glycemic index of the fruits and vegetables you choose. The glycemic index is a measure of how quickly a particular food raises blood sugar levels. Fruits and vegetables with a low glycemic index are ideal for diabetes management, as they provide sustained energy without causing spikes in blood sugar levels.

Preparing Fruits and Vegetables for Juicing

Once you've selected the best fruits and vegetables for juicing, the next step is preparing them for juicing. Proper preparation is essential for getting the most out of your fruits and vegetables and ensuring that your juice is nutrient-dense and delicious.

Start by washing your fruits and vegetables thoroughly under running water. This will help remove any dirt, pesticides, or other contaminants that may be present on the surface.

Next, remove any stems, seeds, or tough outer skins from your fruits and vegetables. These parts can be tough to juice and may produce bitter or unpleasant flavors in your juice.

Finally, chop your fruits and vegetables into small pieces that will fit easily into your juicer. This will help ensure that your juicer can extract as much juice as possible from your fruits and vegetables, and will make the juicing process smoother and more efficient.

In summary, getting started with juicing for diabetes is a simple and straightforward process. By choosing the right juicer, selecting the best fruits and vegetables for juicing, and properly preparing them for juicing, you can create delicious, nutrient-dense juices that can help manage your diabetes and improve your overall health.

Juicing can be a convenient and tasty way to consume a variety of fruits and vegetables that you may not otherwise eat. It can also be a great way to get more fiber and nutrients into your diet without adding a lot of calories.

However, it's important to remember that juicing should not be the only way you consume fruits and vegetables. It's still important to eat a balanced diet that includes a variety of whole foods, including whole fruits and vegetables.

In addition, it's important to monitor your blood sugar levels closely when juicing, as some fruits and vegetables can be high in natural sugars that can cause blood sugar spikes. It's always a good idea to check with your healthcare provider before making any significant changes to your diet or exercise routine.

In the next chapter, we'll explore some of the best juicing recipes for diabetes management, including juices that are high in fiber, low in sugar, and packed with nutrients that can help keep your blood sugar levels stable.

Chapter 3

Essential Nutrients for Diabetes Management

Diabetes management requires a comprehensive approach that includes not only medication and exercise but also a well-balanced diet that provides the essential nutrients that can help keep blood sugar levels in check. Some of the most important nutrients for diabetes management include vitamins, minerals, and antioxidants.

Vitamins play a crucial role in the body's metabolism and can help regulate blood sugar levels. Vitamin C, for example, can help lower blood sugar levels and reduce inflammation, while vitamin D can help improve insulin sensitivity. Other important vitamins for diabetes management include vitamins E, B6, and B12.

Minerals are also essential for diabetes management. Magnesium, for example, can help improve insulin sensitivity and reduce the risk of developing type 2 diabetes. Zinc is another important mineral that can help regulate blood sugar levels and improve insulin sensitivity. Other important minerals for diabetes management include chromium, manganese, and potassium.

Antioxidants are also crucial for diabetes management. These compounds help protect the body from the harmful effects of free radicals, which can damage cells and contribute to chronic diseases like diabetes. Some of the most important antioxidants for diabetes management include vitamin C, vitamin E, beta-carotene, and selenium.

When it comes to juicing for diabetes management, it's important to focus on fruits and vegetables that are particularly rich in these essential nutrients. Some of the best fruits and vegetables for diabetes management include:

- Leafy greens: Leafy greens like spinach, kale, and Swiss chard are packed with essential nutrients like magnesium, potassium, and vitamin K.

- Berries: Berries like blueberries, strawberries, and raspberries are high in fiber, vitamin C, and antioxidants.

- Citrus fruits: Citrus fruits like oranges, grapefruits, and lemons are high in vitamin C and flavonoids, which can help improve insulin sensitivity.

- Cruciferous vegetables: Cruciferous vegetables like broccoli, cauliflower, and Brussels sprouts are high in fiber, vitamin C, and antioxidants.

- Sweet potatoes: Sweet potatoes are high in fiber and antioxidants like beta-carotene, which can help improve insulin sensitivity.

When incorporating these essential nutrients into your juicing routine, it's important to keep in mind that some fruits and vegetables can be high in natural sugars, which can cause blood sugar spikes. It's important to monitor your blood sugar levels closely and choose fruits and vegetables that are low in sugar.

One way to incorporate these essential nutrients into your juicing routine is by creating juices that combine a variety of fruits and vegetables. For example, a juice made from spinach, kale, berries, and citrus fruits can provide a wide range of essential nutrients that can help manage diabetes.

Another way to incorporate these essential nutrients into your juicing routine is by adding supplements like vitamin D, magnesium, or zinc to your juices. These supplements can help fill any nutritional gaps and provide additional support for diabetes management.

In conclusion, incorporating essential nutrients into your juicing routine can be a simple and effective way to manage diabetes and improve overall health. By focusing on fruits and vegetables that are particularly rich in these nutrients and monitoring your blood sugar levels closely, you can create delicious and nutritious juices that support your diabetes management goals.

Chapter 4

Juicing Recipes for Diabetes Management

Juicing can be an excellent way to incorporate more fruits and vegetables into your diet, which can be particularly beneficial for individuals with diabetes. By juicing a variety of nutrient-rich fruits and vegetables, you can create delicious and nutritious drinks that help manage diabetes and boost overall health.

Here are some juicing recipes that are specifically tailored for diabetes management:

1. Green juice:

Ingredients:
- 2 cups spinach
- 1 cucumber
- 1 green apple
- 1/2 lemon
- 1 inch ginger

Instructions:
1. Wash all the ingredients and chop them into smaller pieces.
2. Add them to your juicer and juice.
3. Serve immediately.

This juice is packed with essential nutrients like vitamins, minerals, and antioxidants. Spinach is particularly rich in magnesium and potassium, which can help regulate blood sugar levels. Cucumber is low in sugar and high in fiber, while ginger has anti-inflammatory properties that can help reduce inflammation in the body.

2. Citrus and carrot juice:
Ingredients:

- 2 carrots
- 1 orange
- 1 grapefruit
- 1 inch ginger

Instructions:
1. Wash all the ingredients and chop them into smaller pieces.
2. Add them to your juicer and juice.
3. Serve immediately.

This juice is low in sugar but high in essential nutrients like vitamin C and beta-carotene. The citrus fruits can help improve insulin sensitivity, while the ginger provides anti-inflammatory properties that can help manage diabetes.

3. Beetroot and apple juice:
Ingredients:
- 1 medium-sized beetroot

- 2 green apples
- 1/2 lemon

Instructions:
1. Wash all the ingredients and chop them into smaller pieces.
2. Add them to your juicer and juice.
3. Serve immediately.

This juice is high in essential nutrients like iron, magnesium, and vitamin C. Beetroot is particularly beneficial for diabetes management, as it can help lower blood sugar levels and improve insulin sensitivity. The apples provide a touch of sweetness without adding too much sugar.

4. Carrot and ginger juice:
Ingredients:
- 4 carrots
- 1 inch ginger
- 1/2 lemon

Instructions:
1. Wash all the ingredients and chop them into smaller pieces.
2. Add them to your juicer and juice.
3. Serve immediately.

This juice is packed with essential nutrients like beta-carotene and vitamin C. Carrots are low in sugar but high in fiber, while ginger provides anti-inflammatory properties that can help manage diabetes.

5. Pineapple and cucumber juice:
Ingredients:
- 1 cup chopped pineapple
- 1/2 cucumber
- 1/2 lemon
- 1 inch ginger

Instructions:
1. Wash all the ingredients and chop them into smaller pieces.
2. Add them to your juicer and juice.
3. Serve immediately.

This juice is low in sugar but high in essential nutrients like vitamin C and fiber. Pineapple contains an enzyme called bromelain, which can help reduce inflammation in the body. Cucumber is low in sugar and high in fiber, while ginger provides anti-inflammatory properties that can help manage diabetes.

When creating your own juicing recipes for diabetes management, it's important to focus on fruits and vegetables that are low in sugar but high in essential nutrients like vitamins, minerals, and antioxidants. Be sure to monitor your blood sugar levels closely and make adjustments to your recipes as needed. With a little creativity and experimentation, you can create delicious and nutritious juices that help manage diabetes and boost overall health.

Chapter 5

Creating a Juicing Routine for Diabetes Management

Juicing can be a powerful tool in managing diabetes, but it's important to have a consistent routine to see the best results. In this chapter, we'll discuss tips and strategies for creating a juicing routine that works for you.

Incorporating Juicing into Your Daily Routine

One of the keys to successfully incorporating juicing into your routine is to make it a habit. This means setting aside time each day or week specifically for juicing. Some people prefer to juice in the morning, while others prefer to do it in the evening. The best time to juice is the time that works best for you and your lifestyle.

It's also important to have a designated space for juicing. This can be a corner of your kitchen or a dedicated area on your countertop. Having a dedicated space will make it easier to stay organized and motivated to juice regularly.

Another tip for incorporating juicing into your daily routine is to plan ahead. Decide on the fruits and vegetables you'll use for your juice in advance, so you can make sure you have everything you need on hand. This can also help you stay on track with your diet and avoid unhealthy choices.

When to Juice and How Often

The frequency of juicing depends on personal preferences and health goals. Some people juice every day, while others juice a few times a week. It's important to listen to your body and adjust your routine accordingly.

If you're new to juicing, it's a good idea to start slowly and gradually increase your frequency. This will give your body time to adjust to the new nutrients and avoid any digestive discomfort.

A common question for those with diabetes is whether it's better to juice before or after a meal. The answer to this question depends on your personal preferences and blood sugar levels. Some people find it helpful to juice before a meal to help regulate their blood sugar levels, while others prefer to juice after a meal as a healthy dessert alternative.

Tracking the Effects of Juicing on Blood Sugar Levels

One of the benefits of juicing for diabetes management is its potential to lower blood sugar levels. To track the effects of juicing on your blood sugar, it's important to monitor your levels regularly.

Before starting a juicing routine, take a baseline measurement of your blood sugar levels. You can then track your levels over time to see if there are any changes or improvements. It's important to note that juicing should be used in conjunction with other diabetes management strategies, such as medication and a healthy diet.

Conclusion

Incorporating juicing into your routine can be a powerful tool in managing diabetes. By following the tips and strategies outlined in this chapter, you can create a juicing routine that works for you and helps you reach your health goals. Remember to listen to your body, track your blood sugar levels, and consult with your healthcare provider before making any changes to your diabetes management plan.

Chapter 6

Juicing for Weight Loss and Diabetes Management

Diabetes and weight management are often closely linked, as excess weight can increase the risk of developing type 2 diabetes, and diabetes itself can make it more difficult to lose weight. In this chapter, we'll explore how juicing can be used as part of a healthy weight loss program, while also managing diabetes.

The Link Between Weight Loss and Diabetes Management

Maintaining a healthy weight is important for managing diabetes. Excess weight can increase insulin resistance, making it more difficult for the body to regulate blood sugar levels. Losing weight can help improve insulin sensitivity, making it easier for the body to regulate blood sugar.

However, traditional weight loss methods, such as calorie restriction, can be difficult to maintain and can lead to nutrient deficiencies. Juicing can be a useful tool in weight loss, as it allows you to consume large quantities of fruits and vegetables in a low-calorie form.

Using Juicing as Part of a Healthy Weight Loss Program

Juicing can be a healthy and effective way to lose weight when used in conjunction with a balanced diet and regular exercise. When incorporating juicing into a weight loss program, it's important to focus on creating low-calorie, high-nutrient juices.

One of the keys to using juicing for weight loss is to include a variety of fruits and vegetables in your juices. This not only provides a range of nutrients but also helps to keep your taste buds interested and prevent boredom.

Another important aspect of using juicing for weight loss is to avoid adding high-calorie ingredients, such as sweeteners or fruit juices. Instead, focus on using low-calorie ingredients, such as leafy greens and low-sugar fruits like berries and citrus fruits.

Tips and Tricks for Creating Low-Calorie, High-Nutrient Juices

When creating juices for weight loss and diabetes management, there are a few key tips and tricks to keep in mind. These include:

- Focus on vegetables: Vegetables are low in calories and high in nutrients, making them ideal for weight loss and diabetes management. Aim to include a variety of colorful vegetables in your juices, such as spinach, kale, cucumbers, and celery.

- Use low-sugar fruits: While fruits can be a healthy addition to your juices, some fruits are high in sugar and calories. Opt for low-sugar fruits, such as berries, citrus fruits, and apples.

- Add protein and healthy fats: Protein and healthy fats can help keep you feeling full and satisfied after drinking your juice. Add sources of protein and healthy fats, such as chia seeds, nut butter, or Greek yogurt, to your juices.

- Experiment with herbs and spices: Herbs and spices can add flavor to your juices without adding calories. Try adding ginger, turmeric, or mint to your juices for a boost of flavor and health benefits.

Conclusion

Juicing can be a powerful tool in managing diabetes and promoting weight loss when used in conjunction with a healthy diet and exercise. By focusing on low-calorie, high-nutrient juices and incorporating a variety of fruits, vegetables, and healthy additions, you can create delicious and nutritious juices that support your weight loss and diabetes management goals. Remember to consult with your healthcare provider before making any changes to your diabetes management plan.

Chapter 7

Overcoming Common Juicing Challenges

Juicing for diabetes management can be a highly beneficial and rewarding practice, but it can also come with its fair share of challenges. In this chapter, we will explore some common challenges that may arise when juicing for diabetes management, and provide tips and tricks for overcoming them.

Time Constraints

One of the most common challenges people face when juicing for diabetes management is time constraints. Preparing fresh fruits and vegetables for juicing can be time-consuming, and busy schedules can make it difficult to find the time to juice regularly.

To overcome this challenge, it's important to prioritize juicing as part of your daily routine. Try setting aside specific times of day to juice, such as in the morning before work or in the evening after dinner. You can also try preparing your fruits and vegetables in advance to save time. For example, you can wash and chop your produce ahead of time and store it in the refrigerator until you're ready to juice.

Another option is to invest in a high-quality juicer that can juice quickly and efficiently. Look for juicers with large feeding tubes, which can save time by allowing you to juice whole fruits and vegetables without the need for chopping or peeling.

Budget Concerns

Another challenge that can arise when juicing for diabetes management is budget concerns. Fresh fruits and vegetables can be expensive, and investing in a high-quality juicer can also be a significant expense.

To overcome this challenge, it's important to be strategic in your juicing choices. Look for fruits and vegetables that are in season, as they tend to be less expensive. You can also try shopping at farmers' markets or local produce stands, which may offer lower prices than grocery stores.

In addition, consider purchasing fruits and vegetables in bulk, and freezing them for later use. This can help save money in the long run, while also ensuring that you always have fresh produce on hand for juicing.

Juicer Malfunctions

Another common challenge that can arise when juicing for diabetes management is juicer malfunctions. Juicers are complex machines with many moving parts, and they can sometimes break down or malfunction.

To prevent juicer malfunctions, it's important to invest in a high-quality juicer and to take good care of it. Follow the manufacturer's instructions for cleaning and maintenance, and be sure to clean your juicer after each use to prevent buildup and blockages.

If your juicer does malfunction, don't panic. Most juicers come with a warranty, so you may be able to have it repaired or replaced at no cost. In the meantime, consider using a blender or food processor to create smoothies instead of juices.

Unappetizing Juices

Finally, another common challenge that can arise when juicing for diabetes management is unappetizing juices. Juices that are too bitter or too sweet can be unappealing, and can make it difficult to stick to a juicing routine.

To create more appetizing juices, try experimenting with different combinations of fruits and vegetables. Some fruits and vegetables, such as ginger and lemon, can help balance out bitterness, while others, such as apples and carrots, can add natural sweetness.

In addition, be sure to use fresh, high-quality produce, and to store it properly to maintain freshness. Finally, don't be afraid to add in additional flavorings or spices, such as cinnamon or mint, to create a more appealing taste.

Conclusion

Juicing for diabetes management can come with its fair share of challenges, but with the right tools and techniques, it can also be a highly rewarding and beneficial practice. By prioritizing juicing in your daily routine, being strategic in your product choices, and troubleshooting common juicing challenges, you can create delicious and nutritious juices that help regulate blood sugar levels and improve overall health.

Remember, juicing is just one component of a comprehensive diabetes management plan. It is important to also focus on other lifestyle factors, such as exercise and a healthy diet, and to work closely with your healthcare provider to ensure you are properly managing your condition.

By taking a holistic approach to diabetes management, you can optimize your health and well-being and improve your quality of life. So don't be afraid to experiment with different fruits and vegetables, try new recipes, and find what works best for you and your unique needs. With dedication, patience, and persistence, you can harness the power of juicing to manage your diabetes and enjoy a happier, healthier life.

Chapter 8

Integrating Juicing into a Comprehensive Diabetes Management Plan

Juicing can be a powerful tool in the management of diabetes, but it is just one component of a comprehensive approach to diabetes management. To achieve optimal health and well-being, it is important to also focus on other lifestyle factors, such as exercise, diet, and medication.

In this chapter, we will explore how juicing can be integrated into a comprehensive diabetes management plan, and provide tips and tricks for creating a sustainable and effective plan that includes juicing.

Integrating Juicing into a Comprehensive Diabetes Management Plan

Juicing can be an effective way to supplement a healthy diet, increase nutrient intake, and regulate blood sugar levels. However, it is important to remember that juicing alone is not a comprehensive solution to diabetes management. To achieve optimal health, it is important to also focus on other lifestyle factors, such as exercise and medication.

Here are some tips for integrating juicing into a comprehensive diabetes management plan:

- Work with a Healthcare Provider: Before incorporating juicing into your diabetes management plan, it is important to consult with your healthcare provider. They can help you determine the best way to incorporate juicing into your plan, and provide guidance on how to regulate your blood sugar levels.

- Focus on Nutrient-Dense Foods: When juicing for diabetes management, it is important to focus on nutrient-dense foods that are low in sugar. This includes leafy greens, cruciferous vegetables, and low-glycemic fruits like berries and citrus fruits.

- Incorporate Exercise: Exercise is an important component of diabetes management, as it can help regulate blood sugar levels and improve overall health. Consider incorporating a daily exercise routine into your plan, such as walking, jogging, or strength training.

- Monitor Your Blood Sugar Levels: To effectively manage diabetes, it is important to monitor your blood sugar levels regularly. This will help you identify patterns and adjust your plan as needed.

- Consider Medication: For some individuals with diabetes, medication may be necessary to regulate blood sugar levels. Work with your healthcare provider to determine the best medication regimen for your unique needs.

Creating a Sustainable and Effective Diabetes Management Plan

Incorporating juicing into a comprehensive diabetes management plan can be a highly effective way to regulate blood sugar levels and improve overall health. However, it is important to create a sustainable and effective plan that is tailored to your unique needs.

Here are some tips for creating a sustainable and effective diabetes management plan that includes juicing:

1. Set Realistic Goals: When creating a diabetes management plan, it is important to set realistic goals that are achievable. This may include incorporating juicing into your daily routine, increasing your exercise routine, or monitoring your blood sugar levels regularly.

2. Track Your Progress: Tracking your progress can help you stay motivated and on track with your diabetes management plan. Consider keeping a journal or using a mobile app to track

your juicing habits, exercise routine, and blood sugar levels.

3. Seek Support: Diabetes management can be challenging, so it is important to seek support from friends, family, and healthcare providers. Consider joining a diabetes support group, or working with a registered dietitian or diabetes educator to help you stay on track with your plan.

4. Make Sustainable Changes: To create a sustainable diabetes management plan, it is important to make gradual, sustainable changes to your lifestyle. This may include incorporating one new juicing recipe into your routine each week, or gradually increasing your exercise routine over time.

5. Celebrate Your Successes: Managing diabetes can be challenging, so it is important to celebrate your successes along the way. Take time to acknowledge and celebrate the progress you have made, and use it as motivation to continue working towards your goals.

Conclusion

Incorporating juicing into a comprehensive diabetes management plan can be a highly effective way to manage blood sugar levels, improve overall health, and reduce the risk of complications associated with diabetes. By combining juicing with other lifestyle changes, such as regular exercise, a healthy diet, and medication management, individuals with diabetes can create a well-rounded and sustainable approach to managing their condition.

Remember, juicing is not a replacement for medical treatment, and individuals with diabetes should always consult with their healthcare provider before making any significant changes to their management plan. However, by using the information and tips provided in this book, individuals with diabetes can feel empowered to take an active role in their health and make positive changes to their daily routine.

By understanding the benefits of juicing for diabetes management, selecting the right product, creating delicious and nutritious juices, and integrating juicing into a broader diabetes management plan, individuals with diabetes can take control of their health and improve their overall well-being.

Chapter 9

Juicing Beyond Diabetes Management

Juicing is not just a powerful tool for managing diabetes; it can also promote overall health and wellness. The vitamins, minerals, and antioxidants found in fresh fruits and vegetables can provide a wide range of health benefits, from boosting immunity to improving skin health. In this chapter, we will explore the broader benefits of juicing and provide tips and recipes for using juicing as part of a broader health and wellness routine.

Benefits of Juicing for Overall Health

Juicing can provide a range of benefits for overall health and wellness. Some of the key benefits of juicing include:

- Improved Digestion: Juicing can help to improve digestion by providing the body with essential nutrients in an easily digestible form. The high fiber content of many fruits and vegetables can also promote healthy digestion.

- Increased Energy: The vitamins and minerals found in fresh fruits and vegetables can help to boost energy levels and reduce fatigue.

- Better Immunity: Juicing can provide the body with a range of essential vitamins and minerals that support a healthy immune system, helping to fight off infection and disease.

- Improved Skin Health: The vitamins and antioxidants found in many fruits and vegetables can help to improve skin health and reduce the signs of aging.

- Detoxification: Juicing can help to support the body's natural detoxification processes, helping to remove toxins and waste products from the body.

Recipes for Juices that Promote Overall Health and Wellness

Here are some recipes for juices that promote overall health and wellness:

1. Green Detox Juice: This juice is packed with nutrients and antioxidants that support overall health and wellness.

Ingredients:
- 1 cucumber
- 2 celery stalks
- 1 green apple
- 1 handful of spinach
- 1 handful of kale
- 1/2 lemon

- 1/2 inch piece of ginger

Directions: Wash and chop all ingredients, then juice in a high-quality juicer.

2. Carrot and Orange Juice: This juice is high in vitamin C and antioxidants, which support immunity and overall health.

Ingredients:
- 4 carrots
- 2 oranges
- 1 inch piece of ginger

Directions: Wash and chop all ingredients, then juice in a high-quality juicer.

3. Beet and Berry Juice: This juice is high in antioxidants and anti-inflammatory compounds, which promote overall health and reduce the risk of chronic disease.

Ingredients:
- 1 beet
- 1 cup of mixed berries (such as strawberries, blueberries, and raspberries)
- 1/2 lemon

Directions: Wash and chop all ingredients, then juice in a high-quality juicer.

Tips for Using Juicing as Part of a Broader Health and Wellness Routine

Here are some tips for using juicing as part of a broader health and wellness routine:

1. Incorporate Juicing into a Balanced Diet: Juicing should be used as part of a broader diet that includes a variety of whole foods, including lean protein, healthy fats, and complex carbohydrates.

2. Experiment with Different Recipes: There are countless recipes for healthy and delicious juices, so don't be afraid to experiment and try new combinations of fruits and vegetables.

3. Use High-Quality Produce: Use fresh, organic produce whenever possible to ensure that you are getting the highest quality nutrients.

4. Listen to Your Body: Pay attention to how your body responds to different juices and adjust your routine as needed. If a particular juice causes digestive issues or other symptoms, it may be best to avoid it.

Conclusion

Juicing can provide a range of benefits for overall health and wellness, beyond just managing diabetes. By incorporating a variety of fruits and vegetables into your juicing routine, experimenting with different recipes, and listening to your body's needs, you can create delicious and nutritious juices that promote optimal health and wellbeing.

While juicing is not a cure-all, it can be a powerful tool in a broader approach to health and wellness. By combining juicing with other healthy lifestyle habits such as regular exercise, a balanced diet, and stress management, you can support your body's natural healing and regeneration processes, enhance your immune function, and promote longevity.

When starting a juicing routine, it is important to listen to your body and pay attention to how different juices make you feel. Everyone's body is unique, and what works for one person may not work for another. It is also important to consult with your healthcare provider, particularly if you have any underlying health conditions or are taking any medications.

Incorporating juicing into your daily routine can be a fun and delicious way to support your overall health and wellbeing. Whether you are looking to manage diabetes, lose weight, or simply promote optimal health, there are a variety of juicing recipes and techniques that can help you achieve your goals. By taking the time to learn about the different fruits and vegetables that are particularly beneficial for your health, experimenting with different recipes and techniques, and staying committed to a regular juicing routine, you can enjoy the many benefits of juicing for years to come.

Chapter 10

The Power of Juicing for Diabetes Management

Juicing has been shown to have numerous benefits for managing diabetes and promoting overall health and wellness. By incorporating a variety of fruits and vegetables into your juicing routine, you can create delicious and nutritious juices that help regulate blood sugar levels, promote weight loss, and provide essential nutrients for optimal health.

In this book, we have covered the basics of juicing for diabetes management, including understanding the disease, choosing the right juicer, selecting the best fruits and vegetables, creating juicing recipes, and overcoming common challenges. We have also discussed how juicing can be integrated into a comprehensive diabetes management plan and used to promote overall health and wellness.

One of the most significant benefits of juicing for diabetes management is its ability to regulate blood sugar levels. By choosing fruits and vegetables that are low in sugar and high in essential nutrients, you can create juices that help keep your blood sugar levels in check. Additionally, juicing can help promote weight loss, which is essential for managing diabetes and reducing the risk of complications.

Incorporating juicing into your diabetes management routine may seem daunting at first, but with the right tools and techniques, it can be a highly rewarding and beneficial practice. By prioritizing juicing in your daily routine, being strategic in your produce choices, and troubleshooting common juicing challenges, you can create delicious and nutritious juices that help regulate blood sugar levels and promote overall health.

It's important to remember that juicing is just one piece of the puzzle when it comes to managing diabetes. A comprehensive approach to diabetes management includes exercise, diet, medication, and regular blood sugar monitoring. By incorporating juicing into this broader lifestyle approach, you can create a sustainable and effective diabetes management plan.

In conclusion, juicing has the power to transform your diabetes management routine and promote overall health and wellness. By incorporating the tips and techniques outlined in this book, you can create delicious and nutritious juices that help regulate blood sugar levels, promote weight loss, and provide essential nutrients for optimal health. Remember to consult with your healthcare provider before making any significant changes to your diabetes management plan, and don't hesitate to reach out to resources for further education and support. Here's to your health!

www.ingramcontent.com/pod-product-compliance
Lightning Source LLC
Chambersburg PA
CBHW071028260726
48662CB00024B/2156